Weight Loss Exercise for Women Over 60

Get Fit, Feel Great, and Live Your Best Life

Written by

Emily J. Buckler

DISCLAIMER & POLICIES

This book, "Weight Loss Exercise for Women Over 60: Get Fit, Feel Great, and Live Your Best Life," is here to guide you, but it's not a replacement for your doctor's advice. Always chat with your healthcare professional before starting a new exercise program, especially if you have any health concerns.

We can't be held responsible for any injuries or health problems that might happen from using the information in this book.

Got Questions or Feedback?

We value your thoughts! If you have any questions or feedback about this book, please don't hesitate to reach out. We're always looking for ways to improve and make this resource even better.

Want to Spread the Word?

If you found this book helpful, we'd be incredibly grateful if you recommended it to your friends, family, or anyone else who might benefit from it!

TABLE OF CONTENT

INTRODUCTION

Let's face it, ladies, life after 60 can be incredible. We've gained wisdom, shed anxieties, and maybe even a few bad habits (hopefully!). But sometimes, that wisdom comes with a few unwanted extras – a slower metabolism, a creakier knee, or that stubborn layer around the middle that just won't budge.

Sound familiar? Listen, I've been there. In my early sixties, I found myself staring in the mirror, feeling a disconnect between the vibrant woman I knew I was and the reflection looking back. Sure, life had gotten a little busier with grandkids and volunteer work, but I craved the energy and confidence I used to have.

That's when I embarked on a journey that changed everything – a journey into the world of weight loss exercise specifically designed for women over 60. Let me tell you, it wasn't easy at first. Dusty memories of high-impact aerobics and crash diets came flooding back, leaving me feeling intimidated and overwhelmed. But then, I discovered a whole new world of possibilities, a world where exercise wasn't a punishment, but a celebration of my body's strength and resilience.

This book, my friend, is the culmination of everything I've learned on that journey. It's a roadmap to rediscover the joy of movement, the power of a healthy body, and the confidence that comes with feeling fit and fabulous at any age.

Now, before you start picturing endless hours at the gym or lifting weights that would make Arnold Schwarzenegger sweat, let me assure you, this is different. This book is designed for the real woman, the woman who leads a busy life and doesn't have time for fads or gimmicks. We're talking about exercises you can do at home, with no fancy equipment needed, just your incredible body and a little determination.

What to Expect:
Inside these pages, you'll find a treasure trove of information and support tailored specifically to your needs:

Understanding Your Body: We'll delve into the science behind weight loss after 60, exploring how your body changes and how to optimise your exercise routine for maximum effectiveness.

The Magic of Bodyweight Exercises: Forget expensive gym memberships! This book will unveil the power of bodyweight exercises that sculpt and tone without stressing your joints.

Building a Routine You Love: We'll create a personalised workout plan that fits your schedule and preferences, making exercise a fun and sustainable part of your life.

Fueling Your Body for Success: We'll explore healthy eating habits that support your weight loss goals and nourish your body with the nutrients it needs to thrive.

Staying Motivated: Let's face it, sticking with any program requires a little push. This book will be your cheerleader, offering tips and strategies to keep you inspired and on track.

A Supportive Community: You're not alone in this! We'll explore resources and tools that connect you with other like-minded women on the same journey, creating a network of support and encouragement.

More Than Just Weight Loss:
This book is about so much more than shedding a few pounds. It's about rediscovering the strength and resilience of your body. It's about feeling confident in your own skin and owning your amazing life. It's about having the energy to chase after your dreams, whether it's travelling the world with your besties or simply keeping up with those energetic grandkids.

So, are you ready to embark on this adventure with me? Let's ditch the limitations, embrace the possibilities, and get ready to write the next incredible chapter in your life – a chapter filled with health, vitality, and the confidence that comes with feeling your absolute best!

  Get Fit and Feel Great

PART I:

The Benefits of Bodyweight Exercise for Older Adults

Now, I know what you might be thinking: "Bodyweight exercises? Those won't do much for someone like me." But hold on a sec! Bodyweight exercises can be surprisingly powerful. They help you build strength and muscle, which is fantastic for keeping your bones strong and your metabolism humming along.

CHAPTER 1

Why Bodyweight Exercise is Perfect for You

Let's face it, hitting a certain age can feel like a turning point. The body that once effortlessly kept up with a demanding schedule might start sending different signals. The gym memberships of our youth might lose their lustre, replaced by a yearning for something simpler, more accessible. But the good news is, you don't have to resign yourself to a life of limited movement. In fact, there's a fantastic option waiting for you, right there in your own living room: bodyweight exercise.

Now, before you dismiss it as "too easy" or "not effective enough," hear me out. Bodyweight exercise is a powerful tool for people of all ages, especially those of us who are gracefully entering our golden years. Here's why it might be the perfect fit for you:

Convenience is King: Let's be honest, our schedules can get pretty packed. Between family, work, and social commitments, carving out time for the gym can feel like a luxury. The beauty of bodyweight exercises lies in their simplicity. You don't need a fancy gym membership, expensive equipment, or even a specific location. A sturdy chair, a clear space in your living room, or even a park bench become your personal workout studio. This makes it easier to fit exercise into your day, even if it's just for a quick 15-minute session.

Safety First: As we age, our bodies become more susceptible to injuries. The controlled movements and minimal impact of bodyweight exercises

translate to a safer workout experience. There's no heavy equipment to worry about dropping or awkward manoeuvres that could lead to a fall. You can work at your own pace, gradually increasing difficulty as you gain strength and confidence.

Building Strength for Everyday Life: Don't underestimate the power of your own bodyweight! Squats, lunges, and push-ups, for example, can significantly improve your lower body strength, making it easier to climb stairs, get in and out of chairs, or carry groceries. Upper body exercises like rows and planks can enhance your posture, making you feel taller and more confident. This translates into better balance, coordination, and a reduced risk of falls, promoting greater independence as you age.

Metabolic Boost: Here's a secret: building muscle is key to maintaining a healthy metabolism. Muscle tissue burns more calories at rest than fat tissue, even when you're not actively exercising. Bodyweight exercises, particularly those that focus on major muscle groups, can help you build and maintain muscle mass, giving your metabolism a natural boost.

Mental Wellness Matters: Exercise isn't just about the physical. It's a fantastic way to improve your mood, reduce stress, and boost your overall well-being. Bodyweight workouts can be surprisingly invigorating, releasing endorphins that leave you feeling energised and positive. Regular exercise has also been shown to improve cognitive function and memory, helping you stay sharp and focused.

Variety is the Spice of Life: Bodyweight exercises might sound simple, but there's a surprising amount of variety you can incorporate into your routine. From squats and lunges to planks and push-ups, you can target all the major muscle groups in your body. You can also modify exercises to suit your fitness level, making them more challenging or easier as needed. As you progress, you can explore more advanced variations, keeping your workouts interesting and engaging.

A Journey of Self-Discovery: Most importantly, bodyweight exercise can be a fantastic journey of self-discovery. As you gain strength and build endurance, you'll discover what your body is capable of achieving. It's a chance to celebrate your body's resilience and appreciate its ability to move and adapt. This newfound confidence can spill over into other areas of your life, creating a sense of empowerment that goes beyond the physical.

CHAPTER 2

The Power of Movement

"Staying Active for Improved Health and Well-being"

We've established that bodyweight exercise is a fantastic option for staying active, especially as we enter our golden years. But let's take a step back and delve deeper into the fundamental importance of movement itself. Our bodies are designed to move. Physical activity isn't just about sculpted muscles or weight loss; it's woven into the very fabric of our well-being. Here's how staying active translates into a healthier, happier you!

A Symphony of Systems: Our bodies are intricate systems, with each component relying on the others to function optimally. Movement acts as a conductor, orchestrating a symphony of health benefits. Regular physical activity improves cardiovascular health by strengthening your heart and improving blood flow. This translates into better blood pressure control, reduced risk of heart disease, and increased stamina for everyday activities.

The Metabolic Marvel: Remember how we discussed a healthy metabolism being key to weight management? Well, movement plays a crucial role here too. Exercise helps the body burn calories more efficiently, both during and after your workout. Building muscle further boosts your metabolic rate, making it easier to maintain a healthy weight as you age.

Sugar Blues Be Gone: We all know the dreaded sugar crash after indulging in a sweet treat. Exercise helps regulate blood sugar levels, making you feel more energised throughout the day and reducing cravings for sugary snacks. This can be particularly beneficial for managing conditions like type 2 diabetes.

Strong Bones, Strong Body: As we age, bone density can decrease, leading to a higher risk of osteoporosis and fractures. Weight-bearing exercises, such as squats and lunges, put stress on your bones, stimulating them to become stronger and denser. This helps maintain bone health and reduces the risk of fractures, promoting greater independence and mobility later in life.

The Joint Connection: Regular physical activity can improve the flexibility and lubrication of your joints, making movement smoother and reducing stiffness. This translates into better range of motion, allowing you to perform everyday activities with greater ease and reducing the risk of pain or injury.

Sleep Like a Baby: Ever feel exhausted yet struggle to fall asleep at night? Exercise can be a natural sleep aid. Engaging in physical activity helps regulate your sleep-wake cycle, promoting deeper and more restful sleep. Waking up feeling refreshed and energised sets the stage for a more productive and positive day.

Mental Muscles Matter: The benefits of exercise extend far beyond the physical realm. Regular physical activity has been shown to improve cognitive function, memory, and focus. It can also help reduce symptoms of anxiety and depression, boosting your mood and overall sense of well-being. Exercise releases endorphins, the body's natural feel-good chemicals, leaving you feeling energised and positive.

Social Butterflies Take Flight: Exercise doesn't have to be a solitary pursuit. Joining a group fitness class or walking with a friend can be a fantastic way to stay active and socialise. This can be particularly beneficial for those living alone or facing feelings of isolation. Social interaction keeps you motivated and accountable, while strengthening relationships and providing a sense of belonging.

The Confidence Catalyst: As you gain strength and build endurance through regular exercise, you'll experience a newfound confidence in your body's capabilities. This sense of accomplishment spills over into other areas of your life, creating a positive self-image and a willingness to embrace challenges.

A Life in Motion: Let's face it, life can get overwhelming. But prioritising movement can act as a stress reliever, allowing you to clear your head, de-stress, and gain perspective on challenges. Exercise can be a form of meditation, a chance to focus on your body and connect with yourself in the present moment. This can lead to improved mental clarity and better coping mechanisms for dealing with everyday stressors.

Investing in Your Future: Staying active is truly an investment in your golden years. By prioritising movement, you're laying the foundation for a healthy, independent, and fulfilling future. Exercise helps you maintain your strength and mobility, allowing you to continue living life to the fullest and participating in the activities you love.

CHAPTER 3

Building Strength and Balance for Everyday Activities

Okay, let's get real. As we get older, those everyday tasks that used to be a breeze can start to feel a bit...well, challenging. Reaching for that high shelf in the kitchen cabinet? Suddenly it feels like a mountain climbing expedition. Lugging those heavy grocery bags from the car? More like an Olympic weightlifting event. But fear not, my friends! Bodyweight exercises can be your secret weapon for building strength and balance, making everyday activities feel like a walk in the park (or, shall we say, a stroll through the grocery store!).

Think Strength, Think Superpower: Remember that feeling of accomplishment when you were younger and could effortlessly hoist that heavy suitcase onto the luggage rack? Strength isn't just about aesthetics; it's about empowering your body to tackle daily tasks with confidence. Bodyweight exercises like squats and lunges work wonders for your lower body strength. Imagine carrying those groceries up the stairs feeling like a piece of cake (or maybe a slice of healthy pie?).

Upper Body, Don't Slouch: It's not just your legs that need some love! Upper body exercises like push-ups (modified versions totally count!) and rows can strengthen your arms, shoulders, and back. This translates to better posture, making you feel taller and more confident. Plus, reaching for that jar of spices on the top shelf won't require a precariously balanced step stool anymore.

Balance is Key: Ever feel a little wobbly when reaching for something high up? Balance is crucial as we age, helping to prevent falls and injuries. Bodyweight exercises like single-leg stands and heel-toe walking can improve your sense of balance and stability. Imagine navigating those busy sidewalks like a pro, feeling confident and steady on your feet.

Core Powerhouse: Don't underestimate the importance of your core! Exercises like planks and crunches (with modifications for those with back issues, of course) strengthen your abdominal and back muscles. This core strength acts as your body's internal support system, improving posture, balance, and making everyday movements feel smoother and more effortless.

Everyday Wins, Big and Small: Building strength and balance isn't just about conquering the grocery bags (although that's a pretty awesome victory in itself!). It's about the countless small wins that make a big difference in your daily life. Imagine effortlessly getting out of your favourite chair, playing fetch with your grandkids without getting winded, or gardening with newfound energy.

Variety is the Spice of Life: Bodyweight exercises might sound simple, but there's a surprising amount of variety you can incorporate into your routine. From squats and lunges to planks and wall push-ups, you can target all the major muscle groups in your body, keeping things interesting and challenging. Plus, you can modify exercises based on your fitness level, making them easier or more challenging as needed.

No Gym Required: Here's the beauty of it all – you don't need a fancy gym membership or expensive equipment to build strength and balance. Your own

bodyweight becomes your training tool, and your living room your personal fitness studio. This makes it easy to fit exercise into your day, even if it's just for a quick 15-minute session. Remember, consistency is key! Aim for a few short workouts throughout the week to see steady improvements in your strength and balance.

Start Slow and Celebrate Progress: It's important to listen to your body and start slow, especially if you're new to exercise. Gradually increase the intensity and duration of your workouts as you get stronger. Most importantly, celebrate your progress! Every conquered grocery bag, every achieved repetition of an exercise, is a victory worth acknowledging.

Building strength and balance isn't just about physical benefits; it's about confidence, independence, and a sense of empowerment.

Imagine feeling capable of tackling everyday tasks with ease and grace. Bodyweight exercises can be your key to unlocking that feeling of strength and control, allowing you to embrace life to the fullest and live each day with newfound confidence.

CHAPTER 4

Benefits Beyond the Physical

*"Improved Mood, Memory, and Cognitive
Function"*

We've explored the remarkable physical benefits of bodyweight exercise, from building strength and balance to boosting metabolism and improving bone health. But the power of movement extends far beyond the physical realm, weaving its magic into the very fabric of our mental well-being. Let's delve into the surprising ways bodyweight exercise can enhance your mood, memory, and cognitive function.

The Endorphin Effect: Ever felt that surge of energy and positivity after a good workout? It's not just your imagination! Bodyweight exercise triggers the release of endorphins, natural feel-good chemicals produced by the brain. These endorphins act like tiny messengers, reducing stress hormones and promoting feelings of happiness and well-being. This can significantly improve your mood and leave you feeling more optimistic and energised throughout the day.

Stress Buster Supreme: Let's face it, life can be stressful. But here's the good news: bodyweight exercise can be a powerful tool for managing stress. Physical activity helps regulate the body's stress response system, lowering cortisol levels, the stress hormone. This translates into feeling calmer and more relaxed, promoting mental clarity and better coping mechanisms for dealing with everyday challenges.

The Sleep Connection: A good night's sleep is crucial for both physical and mental health. But let's be honest, sometimes getting those precious Zzz's can feel like an elusive dream. Regular bodyweight exercise can significantly improve sleep quality. Engaging in physical activity helps regulate your sleep-wake cycle, making it easier to fall asleep faster and experience deeper, more restorative sleep. Waking up feeling refreshed and energised sets the stage for a more productive and positive day.

Sharper Mind, Sharper Focus: Studies have shown a strong link between regular physical activity and improved cognitive function. Exercise increases blood flow to the brain, delivering essential oxygen and nutrients that nourish brain cells. This can enhance cognitive skills like memory, focus, and concentration. Engaging in bodyweight exercises can help you feel mentally sharper, improving your ability to learn new things and retain information.

The Creativity Catalyst: Feeling stuck in a rut? Bodyweight exercise can actually spark your creativity! Physical activity increases blood flow throughout the body, including the brain areas associated with creative thinking. This can help you approach problems from new angles and generate fresh ideas. Whether you're brainstorming solutions at work or simply looking to reignite your creative spark, bodyweight exercises can be your secret weapon for a more innovative mind.

Improved Mood, Better Relationships: Let's not underestimate the social and emotional benefits of bodyweight exercise. Joining a group fitness class or exercising with a friend can be a fantastic way to stay active and connect with others. This can be particularly beneficial for those living alone or facing feelings of isolation. Social interaction boosts your mood and sense of belonging, fostering positive relationships and enhancing your overall well-being.

A Sense of Accomplishment: As you gain strength and build endurance through regular bodyweight exercise, you'll experience a newfound sense of accomplishment. This feeling of mastery spills over into other areas of your life, creating a positive self-image and a willingness to embrace challenges. Feeling confident in your body's capabilities can translate into improved self-esteem and a more positive outlook on life.

A Lifelong Investment: The benefits of bodyweight exercise for your mental well-being extend far beyond the immediate effects. By prioritising physical activity, you're investing in your brain health for the long term. Studies have shown that regular exercise can help reduce the risk of cognitive decline and Alzheimer's disease, promoting mental sharpness as you age.

Taking care of your mental well-being is just as important as taking care of your physical health. Bodyweight exercise emerges as a powerful tool for both, offering a convenient and accessible way to boost your mood, memory, and cognitive function. Embrace the power of movement! Make physical activity a regular part of your life and discover the myriad ways it can enhance your mental well-being and overall sense of happiness.

PART II

Getting Started with Bodyweight Exercise

But before I dive headfirst into a million push-ups (wishful thinking!), let's talk about getting started. The good news is, it doesn't require a fancy gym membership or a room full of equipment. Think of your living room as your personal fitness studio!

CHAPTER 5

Safety First

"Essential Considerations Before You Begin"

Enthusiasm is fantastic! You're ready to embrace bodyweight exercise and experience its many benefits. But before you launch into a full-fledged workout routine, let's take a moment to prioritise safety. Here are some essential considerations to keep in mind before you begin:

Start Slow and Gradually Progress: It's easy to get caught up in the excitement and overdo it. But remember, everyone starts somewhere. Begin with low-impact exercises and gradually increase the intensity and duration of your workouts as you get stronger. Consistency is key, so aim for regular short workouts rather than sporadic intense sessions.

Warm-Up and Cool-Down: Never underestimate the importance of a proper warm-up and cool-down routine. A warm-up prepares your body for exercise by increasing blood flow and muscle temperature, while a cool-down helps your body gradually return to its resting state. These simple routines can significantly reduce the risk of injuries. Here's an example:

Warm-Up (5-10 minutes): Light cardio like brisk walking, arm circles, leg swings, gentle stretches. Cool-Down (5-10 minutes): Static stretches for major muscle groups, slow walking, deep breathing exercises.

Proper Form Matters: Performing exercises with proper form is crucial to maximise benefits and minimise the risk of injuries. There are many online resources and exercise tutorials that demonstrate proper form for various bodyweight exercises. This book will also provide detailed instructions and modifications for various exercises. Don't be afraid to ask a fitness professional for guidance if needed.

Focus on Quality Over Quantity: It's not about how many repetitions you can do; it's about doing each one correctly. Focus on maintaining proper form throughout the exercise, even if it means doing fewer repetitions initially. As your strength and endurance improve, you can gradually increase the number of repetitions or sets.

Modify When Needed: Don't be afraid to modify exercises to suit your fitness level or physical limitations. Many bodyweight exercises can be adapted to be easier or more challenging. For example, wall push-ups are a great modification for regular push-ups, and squats can be done without weights if needed.

Hydration is Key: Staying properly hydrated is essential for optimal performance and recovery. Always drink plenty of water before, during, and after your workout. Listen to your thirst cues and adjust your water intake accordingly.

Choose Comfortable Clothing and Supportive Footwear: Wear loose-fitting, comfortable clothing that allows for freedom of movement. If you're exercising on a hard surface, consider wearing supportive shoes to prevent injuries.

Find an Exercise Buddy (Optional): Working out with a friend or family member can be a fantastic way to stay motivated and accountable. Plus, it can add a social element to your exercise routine, making it more enjoyable.

Listen and Learn: There's always more to learn! Utilise online resources, exercise videos, or consider consulting a certified personal trainer for personalised guidance. The more you learn about bodyweight exercise and proper form, the more confident and capable you'll feel in your workouts.

Celebrate Your Progress: It's important to acknowledge and celebrate your achievements, big or small! Every exercise session completed, every milestone reached, is a victory worth celebrating. This will help you stay motivated and keep moving forward on your fitness journey.

By following these essential considerations, you can set yourself up for a successful and enjoyable bodyweight exercise experience. Remember, it's about progress, not perfection. Embrace the journey, listen to your body, and enjoy the amazing benefits of moving your body and feeling your best!

CHAPTER 6

Choosing the Right Exercises for Your Fitness Level

Enthusiasm is high, safety precautions are in place – it's time to delve into the exciting world of bodyweight exercises! But with a multitude of exercises available, how do you choose the right ones for you? Here's where personalization comes in. Selecting exercises that align with your current fitness level is crucial for maximising benefits and minimising the risk of injuries.

Taking Stock: Before diving headfirst into workout routines, take a moment to assess your current fitness level. Are you a complete beginner, someone who occasionally exercises, or do you consider yourself relatively active? Here's a breakdown to help you gauge your starting point:

Beginner: If you're new to exercise or haven't been active for a while, starting slow is key. Opt for low-impact exercises that are gentle on your joints. Examples include bodyweight squats, lunges, wall push-ups, and gentle stretches.

Intermediate: If you have some experience with exercise and a basic level of fitness, you can progress to more challenging bodyweight exercises. Squats with variations, push-ups from the knees, planks, and lunges with arm raises are all fantastic options.

Advanced: For those who are already active and have a strong fitness foundation, the possibilities are even wider. Advanced bodyweight exercises like jump squats, single-leg squats, decline push-ups, and plank variations can provide a significant challenge.

Tailoring Your Routine: Now that you have a sense of your starting point, it's time to personalise your bodyweight exercise routine. Here are some key considerations:

Muscle Groups: Aim to target all the major muscle groups in your body throughout the week. This ensures balanced development of strength and functionality.

Intensity and Duration: Beginners should focus on lower-intensity exercises and shorter workout durations. As your fitness improves, gradually increase the intensity (e.g., adding variations) and duration of your workouts.

Frequency: Consistency is key! Aim for at least 2-3 bodyweight exercise sessions per week, with rest days in between to allow your body to recover.

Building Your Routine: Here are some helpful tools for building your personalised bodyweight exercise routine:

Sample Workouts: This book will provide a variety of sample routines tailored to different fitness levels.

These routines offer a starting point, allowing you to customise them as needed.

Consult a Professional: If you need personalised guidance or have specific limitations, consider consulting a certified personal trainer. They can create a program specifically tailored to your fitness level and goals.

By following the right exercises for your fitness level and incorporating these strategies, you'll create a personalised bodyweight exercise routine that's both effective and enjoyable. This sets you on the path to achieving your fitness goals and experiencing the multitude of benefits bodyweight exercise has to offer. Remember, it's about progress, not perfection. Embrace the journey, celebrate your milestones, and enjoy the process of getting stronger, healthier, and feeling your best!

CHAPTER 7

Warm-Up and Cool-Down Routines to Prepare Your Body

You've chosen the perfect bodyweight exercises for your fitness level, and excitement is brewing. But before you dive into your workout, prioritising proper warm-up and cool-down routines is crucial. These routines act as bookends to your exercise session, preparing your body for activity and promoting optimal recovery.

The Warm-up: Waking Up Your Body:

Think of your warm-up as gently coaxing your body out of a resting state and preparing it for the demands of exercise. Here's why it's important:

Increased Blood Flow: Gentle movements elevate your heart rate and blood flow, delivering essential oxygen and nutrients to your muscles. This prepares them for activity and reduces the risk of injury.

Enhanced Muscle Elasticity: Warm-up movements increase the temperature of your muscles, making them more pliable and less prone to strain or tear.

Improved Joint Mobility: Gentle stretches lubricate your joints and improve their range of motion,

 Get Fit and Feel Great

allowing for smoother and more efficient movement during your workout.

Mental Preparation: A brief warm-up can also act as a mental transition from your day to your workout. It allows you to focus on your body and prepare for the physical activity ahead.

Crafting Your Warm-up:
An effective warm-up should be dynamic, gradually increasing your heart rate and blood flow. Here's a basic structure you can adapt based on your preferences:

5-10 Minutes of Light Cardio: Brisk walking, jumping jacks, or jogging on the spot are fantastic options to elevate your heart rate and get your blood pumping.

Dynamic Stretches: Unlike static stretches, dynamic stretches involve controlled movements that gently stretch your major muscle groups. Examples include arm circles, leg swings, and lunges with twists.

The Cool-down: Winding Down And Recovering:

Your workout doesn't end with the last repetition. A proper cool-down routine allows your body to gradually return to its resting state and promotes optimal recovery. Here's what a cool-down does:

Reduced Muscle Tension: Static stretches held for 20-30 seconds help to lengthen and relax your muscles, reducing post-workout soreness and stiffness.

Improved Blood Flow: Light cardio like walking or gentle yoga poses help to maintain blood flow and remove metabolic waste products produced during exercise.

Gradual Heart Rate Decrease: A cool-down allows your heart rate to gradually return to its resting state, preventing a sudden drop in blood pressure that can cause dizziness.

Mental Transition: The cool-down can also act as a mental transition back to your day, allowing you to unwind and relax after your workout.

Crafting Your Cool-down: An effective cool-down should be low-impact and gradually decrease your activity level. Here's a basic structure you can personalise:

5-10 Minutes of Light Cardio: Continue walking, slow down your jogging on the spot to a gentle stroll, or try some light yoga poses.

Static Stretches: Focus on major muscle groups that were worked during your workout. Hold each stretch for 20-30 seconds and breathe deeply.

The duration and intensity of your warm-up and cool-down will vary depending on the intensity and duration of your workout. For more intense workouts, allow for a longer warm-up and cool-down.

Integrating warm-up and cool-down routines into your bodyweight exercise sessions may seem like an extra step at first. However, by prioritising these routines, you'll be setting yourself up for a more enjoyable and effective workout experience. You'll reduce your risk of injuries, promote faster recovery, and ultimately optimise your results.

The next time you lace up your shoes for a bodyweight exercise session, remember to prime your body for success with a proper warm-up and

wind down with a focused cool-down. Your body
will thank you for it!

CHAPTER 8

Proper Form and Technique for Safe and Effective Workouts

You've crafted a personalised routine, incorporated warm-up and cool-down rituals, and excitement is brimming. But before diving into those bodyweight exercises, let's delve into the critical aspect of proper form and technique. Mastering these elements unlocks the full potential of your workouts, maximising benefits and minimising the risk of injuries.

The Power Of Proper Form:

Think of proper form as the foundation of your bodyweight exercise routine. It ensures you're targeting the intended muscle groups effectively, maximising the results of your efforts. Here's why proper form is crucial:

Muscle Activation: Performing exercises with correct form ensures you're working the intended muscles, leading to more efficient and targeted strength development.

Reduced Injury Risk: Incorrect form can put undue stress on your joints and ligaments, increasing your susceptibility to injuries. Proper form distributes the stress evenly, protecting your body.

Improved Balance and Stability: Many bodyweight exercises inherently enhance balance and stability. When performed with proper form, these benefits are amplified, promoting better coordination and preventing falls.

Movement Efficiency: Mastering proper form allows for smoother and more efficient movement patterns. This translates to better exercise performance and ultimately, more repetitions or sets completed.

Breaking Down Technique:

Technique refers to the specific details of each exercise, including body position, movement execution, and breathing patterns. Here are some key principles to keep in mind:

Maintain a Neutral Spine: Imagine a straight line running through your spine. Aim to maintain this neutral alignment throughout most bodyweight exercises to protect your back.

Engage Your Core: Your core acts as your body's powerhouse. Engaging your core muscles during exercises provides stability and support for your spine and pelvis.

Full Range of Motion: Strive for a full range of motion in each exercise, without compromising proper form. This ensures you're maximising the muscle activation and flexibility benefits.

Controlled Movements: Focus on controlled and deliberate movements, both during the lifting and lowering phases of each exercise. Avoid jerky or ballistic movements that can increase injury risk.

Breathe Properly: Inhale as you prepare to initiate the movement that requires less effort (e.g., lowering yourself during a squat) and exhale as you exert force (e.g., pushing yourself up during a push-up). Proper breathing optimises oxygen delivery and enhances performance.

Learning Proper Form:

There are various resources available to help you master proper form for bodyweight exercises. Here are some suggestions:

Sample Routines in This Book: This book will provide detailed instructions and illustrations for various bodyweight exercises, emphasising proper form.

Practice Makes Perfect:

Mastering proper form takes time and practice. Don't be discouraged if you don't feel perfect right away. Here are some tips to enhance your learning process:

Start with Lighter Weights (if applicable): If you're using bodyweight variations with added weights (e.g., weighted squats), start lighter and prioritise proper form over heavier weights.

Focus on Quality Over Quantity: It's better to perform a few repetitions with perfect form than many repetitions with poor form.

Use a Mirror: Utilise a mirror to observe your body position and ensure you're maintaining proper alignment throughout the exercise.

Listen to Your Body: Pain is a signal. If you experience any pain during an exercise, stop immediately and assess your form. Consult a healthcare professional if necessary.

The road to mastering proper form is a continuous learning process. Embrace the journey, prioritise safety, and don't hesitate to seek guidance when needed. As your technique improves, you'll experience a newfound confidence in your movements and witness the benefits of well-executed bodyweight exercises. By following proper form and technique, you'll transform your bodyweight exercises from basic movements into powerful tools for building strength, improving balance, and achieving your fitness goals. So, take a deep breath, focus on mastering the moves, and get ready to experience the transformative power of bodyweight exercise done right.

PART III

Bodyweight Exercises for All Your Major Muscle Groups

Alright, I'm ready to ditch the gym membership and get moving at home! Bodyweight exercises sound perfect – no fancy equipment needed, just my own body. This book mentions exercises for all my major muscle groups, which is fantastic. I want to build strength everywhere, not just my arms (although toned arms would be a nice bonus!).

CHAPTER 9

Upper Body Exercises

"Building Strength in Your Arms, Shoulders, and Back"

Ready to sculpt a strong and toned upper body? Look no further than these fantastic bodyweight exercises! They target all the major muscle groups in your upper body – arms, shoulders, and back – requiring no equipment and minimal space. Let's get started!

Warm-up (5 Minutes):

Before diving into these exercises, it's crucial to warm up your upper body muscles. Here's a quick routine to get your blood flowing and prepare for movement:

Arm circles (30 seconds forward, 30 seconds backward): Make small circles with your arms, gradually increasing the size of the circles. Reverse direction and repeat.

Shoulder rolls (30 seconds forward, 30 seconds backward): Roll your shoulders forward in a circular motion, then reverse and roll them backward.

Arm swings (30 seconds): Swing your arms back and forth across your body, feeling a gentle stretch in your shoulders and chest.

EXERCISES

1. WALL PUSH-UPS (Modification of Push-Ups): (3 sets of 10-12 repetitions)
Benefits: Targets chest, shoulders, and triceps muscles. Strengthens core for stability.

INSTRUCTIONS:

- Stand facing a wall, with your feet shoulder-width apart and about two feet from the wall.
- Place your hands flat on the wall, slightly wider than shoulder-width apart. Keep your elbows bent and close to your body.
- Engage your core and slowly lower your chest towards the wall, bending your elbows. Aim for a 90-degree angle at your elbows.
- Push back up to the starting position in a controlled manner.

Modification: If regular wall push-ups are challenging, start with your hands positioned higher on the wall (closer to your head) and gradually lower them as your strength improves.

2. CHAIR DIPS (3 sets of 10-12 repetitions)
Benefits: Targets triceps muscles for sculpting and toning. Strengthens shoulders for stability.

INSTRUCTIONS:

- Find a sturdy chair with a stable seat. Sit on the edge of the chair with your hands shoulder-width apart, fingertips gripping the front edge of the seat.
- Scoot your body forward so your feet are flat on the floor, hip-width apart, and slightly behind you.
- Straighten your arms, lifting your body off the chair. Lower yourself down by bending your elbows until your arms reach a 90-degree angle.
- Push back up to the starting position in a controlled manner, engaging your triceps muscles.

Modification: If regular chair dips are challenging, start by performing them with your knees bent and feet flat on the floor. Gradually straighten your legs as you get stronger.

3. BICEP CURLS (using water bottles): (3 sets of 10-12 repetitions per arm)
Benefits: Targets bicep muscles for definition and strength.

INSTRUCTIONS:

- Grab two filled water bottles (or any similar weights) with a comfortable grip.
- Stand tall with your feet shoulder-width apart and core engaged.
- Keep your upper arms close to your body and palms facing forward. Curl the water bottles towards your shoulders, squeezing your biceps muscles at the top.
- Slowly lower the water bottles back down to the starting position, feeling the stretch in your biceps.

Modification: If water bottles are too heavy, start with lighter weights (e.g., canned goods) or perform bodyweight bicep curls with your palms facing up.

4. TRICEP EXTENSIONS (3 sets of 10-12 repetitions)

Benefits: Targets tricep muscles for sculpting and toning.

INSTRUCTIONS:

- Stand tall with your feet hip-width apart and core engaged.
- Hold a water bottle (or similar weight) in one hand behind your head, with your elbow bent and pointing up towards the ceiling.
- Keeping your upper arm stationary, straighten your elbow, extending the water bottle behind your head. Squeeze your tricep muscles at the top of the movement.

- Slowly lower the water bottle back down to the starting position, feeling the stretch in your triceps. Repeat with the other arm.

Cool-Down (5 Minutes):

After completing your upper body exercises, it's essential to cool down and allow your muscles to recover. Here's a quick routine:

Arm stretches (30 seconds each): Raise your arm overhead and gently pull it down towards your back with the other hand. Repeat on the other side. Hold each stretch for 30 seconds.

Chest stretch (30 seconds): Clasp your hands behind your back and gently push your chest forward, feeling a stretch across your chest and shoulders. Hold for 30 seconds.

As you get stronger with these exercises, you can gradually increase the difficulty in a few ways:

Increase repetitions/sets: Once you can comfortably perform 12 repetitions with good form, try increasing the repetitions to 15 or even 18 per set. You can also add an extra set to your workout routine.

Shorter rest periods: Shorten your rest periods between sets by 10-15 seconds. This will increase the intensity of your workout and challenge your muscles further.

Advanced variations: Once you've mastered the basic versions of these exercises, explore advanced variations for an extra challenge. Here are some examples:

Wall pike push-ups: For wall push-ups, elevate your hips slightly by placing your toes on a stable platform (e.g., bench). This increases the difficulty on your chest and shoulders.

 Get Fit and Feel Great

Bench dips: If chair dips are too easy, progress to bench dips. Find two sturdy, parallel surfaces (e.g., benches, boxes) of similar height. Place your hands on the edges and perform dips as described, ensuring your feet are off the ground.

Hammer curls: For bicep curls, hold the water bottles with a neutral grip (palms facing inwards) to target a different portion of your bicep muscles.

Overhead tricep extensions: For tricep extensions, perform them with the water bottle held directly overhead, keeping your arm straight throughout the movement. By following these bodyweight exercises into your routine, you'll be well on your way to building a strong and toned upper body.

CHAPTER 10

Lower Body Exercises

"Strengthening Your Legs and Core
Exercises: Squats, Lunges, Calf Raises, Plank
Variations"

Ready to sculpt strong, toned legs and a rock-solid core? Look no further than these fantastic bodyweight exercises! They target all the major muscle groups in your lower body – quads, hamstrings, calves, and core – requiring no equipment and minimal space. Let's get those legs burning and that core firing!

Warm-up (5 Minutes):

Before diving into these lower body exercises, it's crucial to warm up your leg and core muscles.

Here's a quick routine to get your blood flowing and prepare for movement:

Ankle circles (30 seconds forward, 30 seconds backward): Make small circles with your ankles, gradually increasing the size of the circles. Reverse direction and repeat.

High knees (30 seconds): Run in place, bringing your knees up high towards your chest with each step.

Butt kicks (30 seconds): Run in place, kicking your heels up towards your glutes with each step.

Lunges with arm circles (30 seconds per leg): Step forward with one leg, lowering your body into a

lunge. As you hold the lunge, make small circles with your arms for an added core challenge. Repeat on the other side.

EXERCISES

1. SQUATS (3 sets of 10-12 repetitions)

Benefits: Targets quadriceps, hamstrings, glutes, and core. Strengthens leg muscles for stability and power.

INSTRUCTIONS:

- Stand tall with your feet shoulder-width apart, toes pointed slightly outward. Engage your core and keep your back straight.
- As if sitting back into a chair, bend your knees and lower your hips down towards the ground. Keep your knees tracking over your toes and avoid letting them cave inward.
- Lower yourself until your thighs are roughly parallel to the floor. Hold for a brief moment, then push back up to the starting position using your heels.

Modification: If regular squats are challenging, perform them with a chair behind you. Lower yourself down until you gently tap the chair with your glutes, then push back up.

2. Lunges (3 sets of 10-12 repetitions per leg)
Benefits: Targets quadriceps, hamstrings, glutes, and core. Improves balance and coordination.

INSTRUCTIONS:

- Stand tall with your feet hip-width apart. Step forward with one leg, lowering your body down into a lunge. Your front knee should bend at a 90-degree angle, and your back knee should nearly touch the ground.
- Keep your torso upright and core engaged. Push back up to the starting position using your front heel.
- Repeat lunging forward with the other leg.

Modification: If lunges are challenging, perform walking lunges instead. Take a large step forward with one leg, lower your body into a lunge, then push off with your front foot and step forward with the other leg, continuing the lunge pattern.

3. CALF RAISES (3 sets of 15-20 repetitions)
Benefits: Targets calf muscles for definition and strength. Improves ankle mobility.

INSTRUCTIONS:

- Stand tall with your feet shoulder-width apart. You can perform calf raises on the flat ground, or for an added challenge, find a step or platform.

- Raise yourself up onto your toes, squeezing your calf muscles at the top. Hold for a brief moment, then slowly lower your heels back down to the starting position.

Modification: If performing calf raises on a step or platform is challenging, start by performing them flat-footed.

4. PLANK VARIATIONS (3 sets of holding for 30-60 seconds each)
Benefits: Targets core muscles for stability and strength. Improves posture and balance.

INSTRUCTIONS:

- Get into a high plank position: forearms on the ground, shoulder-width apart, elbows directly under your shoulders, body in a straight line from head to heels. Engage your core and glutes to keep your body stable.

- Hold this position for 30-60 seconds, or as long as you can maintain good form.

PLANK VARIATIONS:

Once you've mastered the basic plank, explore these variations for an extra core challenge:

Side plank: Lie on your side with one forearm on the ground, directly under your shoulder. Stack your feet on top of each other, or stagger them for added stability. Lift your hips off the ground, forming a straight line from head to heels. Hold for 30-60 seconds per side.

High plank with arm raises: Perform a high plank as described above. Raise one arm off the ground, reaching towards the ceiling. Hold for a few seconds, then lower your arm back down and repeat with the other arm. Continue alternating arm raises throughout the plank hold.

Cool-Down (5 Minutes):

After completing your lower body exercises, it's essential to cool down and allow your muscles to recover. Here's a quick routine:

Quad stretch (30 seconds each leg): Stand tall and hold onto something sturdy for balance. Reach back and grab one foot behind your calf. Gently pull your heel towards your glutes, feeling the stretch in your quadriceps. Hold for 30 seconds, then repeat on the other leg.

Hamstring stretch (30 seconds each leg): Sit on the floor with one leg extended straight in front of you. Lean forward, reaching towards your toes with both hands. Feel the stretch in your hamstrings. If you can't reach your toes, hold onto a strap or towel for assistance. Hold for 30 seconds, then repeat on the other leg.

Calf stretch (30 seconds each leg): Stand facing a wall with your hands flat on the wall at shoulder height. Step back one leg, keeping your front heel flat on the ground. Lean into the wall, feeling the stretch in your calf muscle. Hold for 30 seconds, then repeat on the other leg.

As you get stronger with these exercises, you can gradually increase the difficulty in a few ways:

Increase repetitions/sets: Once you can comfortably perform 12 repetitions of squats or lunges with good form, try increasing the repetitions to 15 or even 18 per set. You can also add an extra set to your workout routine.

Hold planks for longer: As planks become easier to hold, challenge yourself by gradually increasing the hold time by 5-10 seconds per set.

Weighted variations: Once you've mastered the bodyweight versions of these exercises, consider adding weight for an extra challenge. Here are some examples:

Weighted squats: Hold a dumbbell or weighted backpack in front of your chest while performing squats.

Weighted lunges: Hold dumbbells in each hand while performing lunges.

Weighted calf raises: Perform calf raises while holding a dumbbell in each hand.

Celebrate your progress, and get ready to feel the burn in the best way possible! Now that you've explored exercises for both your upper and lower body, you're well-equipped to design a complete bodyweight workout routine. Stay tuned for the next chapter, where we'll delve into crafting personalised routines to fit your fitness goals!

CHAPTER 11

Core Exercises

"Strengthening Your Abdominal and Back Muscles for Stability

Your core – the powerhouse of your body – deserves some serious attention! It encompasses all the muscles that support your spine and pelvis, playing a crucial role in stability, balance, and posture. Strengthening your core not only improves your overall fitness but also helps prevent back pain and injuries. In this chapter, we'll explore fantastic bodyweight core exercises that require no equipment and minimal space. Let's fire up those abdominals and build core confidence!

Warm-up (5 Minutes):

Before diving into these core exercises, it's crucial to warm up your core muscles and prepare your body for movement. Here's a quick routine to get your blood flowing and muscles activated:

Pelvic tilts (10 repetitions forward, 10 repetitions backward): Stand tall with your feet shoulder-width apart. Gently tilt your pelvis forward, arching your lower back slightly. Hold for a second, then return to the starting position. Repeat by tilting your pelvis backward, tucking your tailbone under. Hold for a second, then return to the starting position.

Cat-Cow (10 repetitions): Start on all fours with your hands shoulder-width apart and knees hip-width apart. As you inhale, arch your back and look up (cow pose). As you exhale, round your back and tuck your chin to your chest (cat pose). Flow smoothly between these movements.

Spinal twists (10 repetitions each side): Sit on the floor with your knees bent and feet flat on the ground. Engage your core and gently twist your torso to one side, looking over your shoulder. Hold for a second, then return to the starting position. Repeat on the other side.

EXERCISES:

1. CRUNCHES (modifications provided): (3 sets of 10-12 repetitions)**
Benefits: Targets abdominal muscles for definition and strength. Improves core stability.

INSTRUCTIONS:

- Lie on your back with your knees bent and feet flat on the floor. Place your fingertips lightly behind your head, keeping your elbows pointed out to the sides.

- Engage your core and lift your upper back off the ground, initiating the movement with your abs, not your neck.
- Inhale as you lower back down to the starting position, exhale as you crunch up. Avoid pulling on your neck with your hands.

Modified crunch: If regular crunches cause discomfort in your neck, perform modified crunches. Lie on your back with your knees bent and feet flat on the floor. Cross your arms over your chest and engage your core to lift your upper back slightly off the ground. Lower back down with control.

2. DEAD BUGS (3 sets of 10 repetitions per side)
Benefits: Targets deep core muscles for improved stability and coordination. Strengthens lower back.

INSTRUCTIONS:

- Lie on your back with your knees bent and feet flat on the floor. Extend your arms straight up towards the ceiling.

- Engage your core and slowly lower one arm and the opposite leg down towards the ground, keeping your lower back pressed into the floor. Don't let your back arch.

- Hold for a brief moment, then return to the starting position with control. Repeat by lowering the other arm and opposite leg.

Modified dead bugs: If lowering both an arm and leg at the same time is challenging, start by performing modified dead bugs. Lower just one arm or leg at a time, maintaining a neutral spine throughout the movement.

3. **BIRD-DOGS** (3 sets of 10 repetitions per side)

Benefits: Targets core muscles for stability and coordination. Improves balance and posture.

INSTRUCTIONS:

- Start on all fours with your hands shoulder-width apart and knees hip-width apart. Engage your core and keep your back flat.
- Extend one arm straight out in front of you and the opposite leg straight out behind you, keeping your back parallel to the floor.
- Hold for a brief moment, then return to the starting position with control. Repeat by extending the other arm and opposite leg.

Cool-Down (5 Minutes):

After completing your core exercises, it's essential to cool down and allow your muscles to recover. Here's a quick routine:

Lower back stretch (30 seconds): Lie on your back with your knees bent and feet flat on the floor. Gently hug your knees to your chest and hold for 30 seconds.

Knee rolls (10 repetitions each direction): Lie on your back with your knees bent and feet flat on the floor. Slowly roll your knees from side to side, keeping your shoulders pressed into the ground.

Spinal twists (10 repetitions each side): Lie on your back with your knees bent and feet flat on the floor. Gently lower both knees to one side, keeping your shoulders on the ground. Look over your opposite

shoulder and hold for a second. Repeat on the other side.

As you get stronger with these exercises, you can gradually increase the difficulty in a few ways:

Increase repetitions/sets: Once you can comfortably perform 12 repetitions of crunches (or modified crunches), dead bugs, or bird-dogs with good form, try increasing the repetitions to 15 or even 18 per set. You can also add an extra set to your workout routine.

Hold for longer: For dead bugs and bird-dogs, as holding the extended positions becomes easier, challenge yourself by gradually increasing the hold time by 2-3 seconds per set.

Weighted variations: Once you've mastered the bodyweight versions of these exercises, consider adding weight for an extra challenge. Here are some examples:

Weighted crunches: Hold a weight plate (or water bottle) against your chest while performing crunches.

Weighted dead bugs: Hold a light weight (dumbbell or water bottle) in the extended hand while performing dead bugs.

Weighted bird-dogs: Hold a light weight (dumbbell or water bottle) in the extended hand or leg while performing bird-dogs.

Now that you've explored exercises for all your major muscle groups – upper body, lower body, and core – you're well-equipped to design a complete bodyweight workout routine tailored to your fitness goals. The next chapter will delve into crafting personalised routines, helping you unlock your full potential and achieve peak fitness!

CHAPTER 12

Balance and Flexibility Exercises

"Improving Stability and Range of Motion Exercises: Single Leg Stands, Heel-Toe Walking, Arm Circles, Shoulder Rolls"

Ready to enhance your balance, coordination, and flexibility? Look no further than these fantastic bodyweight exercises! They target your entire body, improving your range of motion and overall movement efficiency. Remember, a balanced and flexible body is a happy (and less injury-prone) body! Let's get moving and embrace the flow.

Warm-up (5 Minutes):
Before diving into these balance and flexibility exercises, it's crucial to warm up your muscles and

prepare your body for movement. Here's a quick routine to get your blood flowing and increase your range of motion:

Neck rolls (10 repetitions each direction): Slowly roll your head in a circular motion, starting forward and then backward. Repeat 10 times in each direction.

Arm circles (10 repetitions forward, 10 repetitions backward): Make small circles with your arms, gradually increasing the size of the circles. Reverse direction and repeat.

Torso twists (10 repetitions each side): Stand with your feet shoulder-width apart and arms outstretched to the sides. Gently twist your torso to

one side, looking over your shoulder. Hold for a second, then return to the starting position. Repeat on the other side.

Leg swings (10 repetitions forward and backward each leg): Stand tall and hold onto something sturdy for balance. Swing one leg forward and backward, keeping your leg straight. Repeat 10 times with each leg.

EXERCISES

1. SINGLE LEG STANDS (3 sets of 30-60 seconds each leg)
Benefits: Improves balance and coordination. Strengthens core and leg muscles for stability.

INSTRUCTIONS:

- Stand tall with your feet hip-width apart. Engage your core and slowly lift one leg off the ground, keeping it straight or slightly bent.
- Focus on a point in front of you for better balance. Hold this position for 30-60

seconds, or as long as you can maintain good form.

- Slowly lower your raised leg back down to the starting position and repeat by standing on the other leg.

Modified single leg stands: If balancing on one leg is challenging, perform modified single leg stands with your arms outstretched to the sides or holding onto something sturdy for support.

2. HEEL-TOE WALKING (3 sets of 30 seconds each direction):
Benefits: Improves balance and coordination. Enhances ankle mobility and flexibility.

INSTRUCTIONS:

- Stand tall with your feet hip-width apart. Take a small step forward, placing your heel down first, followed by your toes.

- Focus on a point in front of you for better balance. Continue taking small heel-toe steps forward for 30 seconds.
- Turn around and walk backward for another 30 seconds, placing your toes down first, followed by your heel.

3. ARM CIRCLES (3 sets of 10 repetitions forward, 10 repetitions backward each direction): Benefits: Improves shoulder mobility and flexibility. Increases range of motion in the upper body.

INSTRUCTIONS:
- Stand tall with your feet hip-width apart and arms extended out to your sides at shoulder height.

- Make small circles with your arms, gradually increasing the size of the circles. Breathe smoothly throughout the movement.

- Reverse direction and repeat, making small circles backward with your arms for 10 repetitions.

4. SHOULDER ROLLS (3 sets of 10 repetitions forward, 10 repetitions backward):
Benefits: Improves shoulder mobility and flexibility. Promotes better posture.

INSTRUCTIONS:

- Stand tall with your feet hip-width apart and arms relaxed at your sides.
- Gently roll your shoulders forward in a circular motion, feeling a stretch in your chest and shoulders.
- Reverse direction and roll your shoulders backward in a circular motion. Breathe smoothly throughout the movement.

Cool-Down (5 Minutes):

After completing your balance and flexibility exercises, it's essential to cool down and allow your muscles to relax and lengthen. Here's a quick routine to improve your overall flexibility:

Hamstring stretch (30 seconds each leg): Sit on the floor with one leg extended straight in front of you. Lean forward, reaching towards your toes with both hands. Feel the stretch in your hamstrings. If you can't reach your toes, hold onto a strap or towel for assistance. Hold for 30 seconds, then repeat on the other leg.

Quad stretch (30 seconds each leg): Stand tall and hold onto something sturdy for balance. Reach

back and grab one foot behind your calf. Gently pull your heel towards your glutes, feeling the stretch in your quadriceps. Hold for 30 seconds, then repeat on the other leg.

Calf stretch (30 seconds each leg): Stand facing a wall with your hands flat on the wall at shoulder height. Step back one leg, keeping your front heel flat on the ground. Lean into the wall, feeling the stretch in your calf muscle. Hold for 30 seconds, then repeat on the other leg.

Neck stretches (10 seconds each side): Gently tilt your head to one side, bringing your ear towards your shoulder. Hold for 10 seconds, then repeat on the other side.

As you improve your balance and flexibility with these exercises, you can gradually increase the difficulty in a few ways:

Increase hold times: For single leg stands and arm circles, as holding these positions becomes easier, challenge yourself by gradually increasing the hold time by 5-10 seconds per set.

Weighted single leg stands: Once you can comfortably balance on one leg for 30 seconds, try holding a light weight (dumbbell or water bottle) in your hand while performing single leg stands.

Advanced walking variations: Explore more challenging walking variations like walking on your tiptoes or walking on your heels to further improve balance and ankle mobility.

Yoga poses: As your flexibility improves, consider incorporating yoga poses into your routine for a more comprehensive flexibility workout.

Now that you've explored a variety of bodyweight exercises targeting different muscle groups and aspects of fitness, you're ready to design a personalised workout routine. The next chapter will delve into crafting workout plans to fit your specific goals and preferences, helping you unlock your full potential and achieve lasting results!

PART IV

Creating Your Personalised Exercise Routine

Alright, champions! We've talked about bodyweight workouts, explored different activities, and hopefully ignited a fitness fire within you. But before you dive headfirst into endless workout plans, let's talk about creating a personalised routine – your very own fitness blueprint!

CHAPTER 13

Designing a Safe and Effective Workout Plan

Ready to unleash your inner fitness start with a month-long bodyweight challenge? This chapter will guide you through designing a safe and effective 31-day workout plan using the entire exercise repertoire you've explored in this book. Let's craft a routine that keeps things interesting, challenges you progressively, and delivers results!

Planning Your Month-Long Challenge:

Here's a step-by-step approach to creating your personalised 31-day bodyweight workout plan:

STEP 1: REVIEW YOUR GOALS:

Revisit your fitness goals established in Chapter 12. Are you aiming for strength, toning, improved flexibility, or overall fitness? This will influence the exercise selection and intensity throughout the month.

STEP 2: STRUCTURE YOUR WEEK:

Divide your week into workout days and rest days. Aim for at least 2-3 workouts per week, with rest days strategically placed for optimal recovery between sessions. Consider factors like your schedule and fitness level when designing your weekly structure. Here's an example:

Option 1: Monday, Wednesday, Friday (workouts) - Tuesday, Thursday, Saturday, Sunday (rest)

Option 2: Monday, Wednesday, Saturday (workouts) - Tuesday, Thursday, Friday, Sunday (rest)

STEP 3: CREATE A FOUR-WEEK WORKOUT ROTATION:

To keep things fresh and avoid plateaus, design a four-week workout rotation. Each week will have a slightly different focus, incorporating exercises from all chapters while gradually increasing intensity. Here's a sample four-week rotation template:

WEEK 1: BUILDING A FOUNDATION

Focus on proper form and mastering the basic bodyweight exercises from Chapters 9-12. Utilise lower repetitions (8-10 reps) with more sets (3-4 sets) to build a solid foundation.

WEEK 2: STRENGTH & TONE

Increase the intensity by incorporating higher repetitions (12-15 reps) with the same number of sets (3-4 sets) or add weighted variations (e.g., holding water bottles) for some exercises.

WEEK 3: POWER UP!

Push your limits with higher intensity workouts. Utilise shorter rest periods (15-30 seconds) between sets, explore HIIT variations (high-intensity interval training), or introduce more challenging exercise variations.

WEEK 4: ACTIVE RECOVERY & FLEXIBILITY

Dedicate this week to active recovery and improved flexibility. Focus on lighter exercises or bodyweight cardio on workout days. Prioritise stretching and mobility exercises throughout the week. This allows your body to recover while maintaining some level of activity.

STEP 4: SAMPLE DAILY WORKOUT EXAMPLES:

Week 1 (Building a Foundation)

Day 1 (Upper Body & Core):

- Warm-Up (5 minutes)

Circuit 1 (3 sets of 8-10 repetitions per exercise):

- Wall Push-Ups
- Chair Dips
- Bicep Curls (using water bottles)
- Tricep Extensions (overhead or behind the head)
- Plank (3 sets of 30 seconds hold)
- Crunches (modifications provided) (3 sets of 10-12 repetitions)
- Cool-Down (5 minutes)

Day 2 (Lower Body & Core):

- Warm-Up (5 minutes)

Circuit 2 (3 sets of 8-10 repetitions per leg):**

- Squats
- Lunges
- Calf Raises (3 sets of 15-20 repetitions)
- Side Plank (3 sets of 30 seconds hold per side)
- Dead Bugs (3 sets of 10 repetitions per side)
- Cool-Down (5 minutes)

Day 3 (Rest)

Repeat Day 1 and Day 2 workouts for the rest of the week, substituting rest days as needed.

Week 2 (Strength & Tone) will follow the same structure with adjustments:

- Increase repetitions to 12-15 per exercise.
- Consider holding weights (water bottles) for some exercises.

- Shorten rest periods slightly (15-20 seconds) between sets.

Week 3 (Power Up!) will again follow the same structure with adjustments:

- Utilise HIIT variations: Perform exercises for 30 seconds each with 15 seconds rest between exercises. Repeat the circuit 3 times.
- Introduce more challenging exercise variations (e.g., single leg squats, advanced plank variations).
- Shorten rest periods further (10-15 seconds) between sets.

Week 4 (Active Recovery & Flexibility):**

- Focus on lighter exercises or bodyweight cardio on workout days (e.g., brisk walking, jumping jacks, bodyweight cardio variations).

- Dedicate a significant portion of your workout time to stretching and mobility exercises from Chapter 12.
- Consider incorporating yoga or Pilates routines specifically designed for flexibility and recovery.
- Prioritise proper sleep and healthy eating habits throughout the week to optimise recovery.

Remember: This is just a sample template. Feel free to adjust it based on your preferences, fitness level, and available time. The key is to create a plan you can realistically stick with and enjoy!

Staying Safe and Effective:
Here are some crucial safety tips to ensure your 31-day challenge is both safe and effective:

Warm-Up and Cool-Down: Never skip the warm-up and cool-down routines. These prepare your body for exercise and promote recovery, respectively.

Proper Form: Pay close attention to form during each exercise. It's better to perform fewer repetitions with good form than many repetitions with improper form, which can lead to injuries.

Listen to Your Body: Don't push yourself beyond your limits. Take rest days when needed, and stop any exercise that causes pain.

Hydration and Nutrition: Stay hydrated by drinking plenty of water throughout the day. Fuel your body with nutritious foods to support your workouts and recovery.

Consult a Healthcare Professional: If you have any pre-existing health conditions, consult a healthcare professional before starting a new exercise routine.

THE FINAL PUSH:

With a well-designed plan, dedication, and consistency, your 31-day bodyweight challenge can be a rewarding and transformative experience. Remember, celebrate your progress, big or small, and enjoy the journey towards a healthier and fitter you!

Congratulations! You've now completed this comprehensive guide to bodyweight exercises and workout plan creation. With the knowledge you've gained, you're well-equipped to design a personalised routine that fits your goals and unleashes your inner fitness star!

CHAPTER 14

Progression And Challenges

"Gradually Increasing Intensity for Continued Improvement"

Alright, folks, buckle up! We're a month into this bodyweight challenge, and let me tell you, it's been a wild ride. Remember how excited I was about those wall push-ups at the beginning? Now, I'm feeling the burn with incline push-ups, and my triceps are screaming (in a good way, I think!). This chapter is all about progression – how to keep pushing yourself and avoid plateaus in your fitness journey. Get ready for some real talk about challenges, victories, and everything in between!

The first few weeks were tough, but they were also incredibly rewarding. I mastered those basic exercises, learned proper form (which is key!), and felt my body getting stronger. But then, something happened – the workouts started feeling...well, predictable. Squats weren't so scary anymore, lunges became a breeze (well, almost!), and those initial wall push-ups? They felt like child's play. That's when I realised the magic word in this whole bodyweight thing: progression.

Chapter 13 talked about creating a four-week workout rotation, and let me tell you, it was a lifesaver! Suddenly, my workouts weren't just about going through the motions. Week Two brought on the "Strength & Tone" phase, upping the repetitions and introducing weighted variations (water bottles became my new best friends!). Those extra reps pushed me further, and held those water bottles during bicep curls? Let's just say my arms were sore in the best way possible. It was a whole new level of challenge, and frankly, it felt awesome!

Week Three was a beast. HIIT variations? Sign me up! Thirty seconds of jumping jacks followed by 15 seconds of rest – repeat three times? Let's do this! My heart rate was sky-high, my lungs were burning, but I pushed through. This high-intensity approach had me sweating like never before, and let me tell you, the endorphin rush afterwards was incredible. It was about pushing my limits, and guess what? Those limits turned out to be further than I thought.

Of course, it wasn't all sunshine and rainbows. There were days when dragging myself out of bed for a workout felt impossible. My muscles were aching, my energy levels were low, and the thought of another round of lunges made me groan. But then I remembered the progress I'd made, the strength I'd gained, and the newfound confidence I felt. Those were the days I relied heavily on the "Listen to Your Body" tip from the book. Sometimes, a rest day was exactly what I needed to come back stronger and tackle the next workout head-on.

Speaking of challenges, let's talk about form! It's easy to get caught up in the reps and sets, forgetting about proper form. I definitely had those days where fatigue would trick me into sacrificing form for an extra push-up. But remember, bad form can lead to injuries, and that's the last thing we want! So, I learned to slow down, focus on my movements, and prioritise quality over quantity. Trust me, the frustration of a missed rep is way better than dealing with an injury that sidelines you.

Here's the thing about progression – it's not always about adding weight or reps. Sometimes, it's about exploring new exercise variations. Take Week Four, for example. The focus shifted to active recovery and flexibility. While I still did some bodyweight cardio and lighter exercises, a big chunk of the workout time was dedicated to stretching and mobility routines. These exercises weren't as intense, but they were crucial! Stretching helped me improve my range of motion, while mobility exercises kept my joints feeling happy. It was all about maintaining a healthy balance and giving my body the TLC it needed to recover and keep improving.

Looking back on this month-long journey, it's been an eye-opener. I've learned that consistency is key – showing up and putting in the effort, even on days when motivation feels low. I've discovered the importance of listening to my body, respecting my limits, and knowing when to take a well-deserved rest day.   And most importantly, I've learned to embrace the challenge! Pushing myself beyond my comfort zone has been incredibly rewarding. Those extra reps, those heavier weights, those HIIT workouts – they've all contributed to my progress, making me stronger, leaner, and more confident than ever before.

So, my fellow bodyweight enthusiasts, here's the takeaway: Don't be afraid to progress! Whether it's adding weight, increasing reps, exploring new variations, or simply focusing on flexibility

CHAPTER 15

Staying Motivated and Making Exercise a Habit

Alright, folks, we've conquered a month of bodyweight workouts, pushed our limits, embraced the challenge, and (hopefully) witnessed some amazing progress. But let's be honest, staying motivated and making exercise a long-term habit can be tough. Life throws curveballs, schedules get hectic, and sometimes, that couch just seems way too inviting after a long day. So, this chapter is dedicated to all the things that can help you keep the fitness flame alive and turn those workouts into a routine you actually enjoy!

First things first, let's talk about the power of "setting realistic goals". We all dream of having washboard abs and sculpted arms overnight, but let's face it, that's not how it works (unless you have a time machine, in which case, can I come along?). Setting achievable goals helps you stay motivated. Remember those first wall push-ups? They felt like a mountain to conquer, but achieving that goal fueled my desire to keep going. Maybe your goal is to master regular push-ups, increase your squat depth, or hold a plank for a longer duration. Whatever it is, set SMART goals – Specific, Measurable, Achievable, Relevant, and Time-bound. Track your progress in a journal, celebrate your wins, and watch your motivation soar!

Now, life happens. There will be days when your schedule gets thrown off, or you just don't feel like tackling a full-blown workout. That's where the concept of **micro-workouts** come in. Don't let a busy day derail your entire fitness routine! Even a quick 10-minute burst of exercise is better than nothing. Squeeze in some squats during your lunch break, do some lunges while waiting for the kettle to boil, or throw in a plank series while watching your favourite show. These micro-workouts might not be your most intense sessions, but they keep your body moving and maintain consistency, which is crucial for building a sustainable habit.

Speaking of consistency, let's talk about the power of **habit stacking**. This is where you link your workout routine to an existing habit you already do regularly. For example, if you always brush your teeth in the morning, try doing a few bodyweight exercises right after. The act of brushing your teeth becomes a trigger for your workout, making it easier to stick to the routine. Similarly, you could do some stretches or bodyweight cardio right before you settle in for the night. By associating your workouts with established habits, you increase the chances of them sticking.

Let's not forget the importance of "finding activities you actually enjoy". Yes, exercise can be challenging, but it shouldn't feel like a punishment! If you hate traditional workouts, explore different bodyweight exercise variations. Maybe dance fitness is more your style, or perhaps bodyweight circuits with a friend keep you engaged. There are endless possibilities! Find activities that spark joy and make you look forward to moving your body. When exercise becomes something you enjoy, it's much easier to stick with it in the long run.

Now, here's a secret weapon: "enlist a workout buddy". Having someone by your side can be a game-changer. A friend can hold you accountable, push you to try harder, and make workouts more fun. You can motivate each other, celebrate milestones together, and commiserate on those tough days. Plus, having someone to rely on helps prevent those dreaded workout bailouts. So, grab a friend, family member, or even a workout buddy online, and make those sweat sessions a team effort!

But what if the motivation monster still rears its ugly head? That's where the power of "positive self-talk" comes in. Dwelling on negative thoughts like "I can't do this" or "I'm not strong enough" will only hinder your progress. Instead, replace those thoughts with positive affirmations like "I can do anything I set my mind to" or "My body is getting stronger every day." Focus on how good you feel after a workout, the progress you've made, and the overall benefits of exercise for your physical and mental health. Believe in yourself, celebrate your achievements, and watch your motivation soar!

Remember, progress isn't always a straight line. There will be days when you feel like a rockstar, and others where you struggle to get through a simple routine. Don't let setbacks define you! "Embrace the journey", celebrate small victories, and enjoy the process. Focus on how much stronger, more confident, and more energised you feel with every workout. It's about making exercise a part of your lifestyle, not just a means to an end

CHAPTER 16

Listen to Your Body

"Recognizing Pain and Knowing When to Rest"

This whole bodyweight challenge has been amazing, but it's also taught me a valuable lesson: the importance of listening to your body. Sure, pushing my limits and seeing progress is incredibly rewarding, but there's a fine line between challenging yourself and pushing things too far. This chapter is all about recognizing pain, knowing when to rest, and making recovery an essential part of the journey.

Remember Week Three of the challenge? The one with HIIT variations? Yeah, that week was intense. Jumping jacks, lunges, mountain climbers – my heart rate was sky high, and I was pushing myself to my absolute limit. Honestly, it felt incredible – that rush of endorphins, the feeling of accomplishment... pure fitness bliss! However, the next day, something felt different. My muscles weren't just sore, they were achy in a way that felt different from the usual post-workout soreness. There was a dull pain in my right knee, and every time I bent it, it sent a jolt of discomfort shooting up my leg.

That's when the lesson of listening to my body hit me hard. Ignoring the pain and pushing through another workout might have felt "tough," but deep down, I knew it wasn't the right thing to do. So, I took a rest day. And then another one. It wasn't easy. There was a part of me that felt guilty for taking a break, like I was somehow failing the challenge. But then I remembered – this challenge wasn't about pushing myself to the point of injury. It was about building a sustainable workout routine, one that respected my body's needs for rest and recovery.

So, I spent those rest days focusing on recovery strategies. I stretched religiously, using the stretches from Chapter 12 to improve my flexibility and loosen up those tight muscles. I also invested in a foam roller, and let me tell you, those self-myofascial release sessions were a lifesaver! Rolling out the tightness in my legs and glutes did wonders for easing the pain and improving my range of motion.

Hydration became another key player in my recovery game.   Drinking plenty of water throughout the day helped flush out toxins and

 Get Fit and Feel Great

promote muscle repair. And guess what? The healthy eating habits I'd adopted during the challenge also played a role. Fueling my body with nutritious foods provided it with the building blocks it needed to heal and recover properly.

Slowly but surely, the pain in my knee started to subside. With each passing day, the dull ache morphed into a manageable tightness. Finally, after a few days of rest and recovery, I cautiously ventured back into my workout routine. This time, I listened even more intently to my body's signals. I modified exercises that caused any discomfort, reduced the intensity, and focused on proper form over pushing myself to the limit.

This experience taught me a valuable lesson: rest isn't a sign of weakness – it's a sign of strength. Taking the time to recover allows your body to repair itself, rebuild muscle tissue, and come back stronger than before. Pushing through pain can lead to injuries, setbacks, and ultimately, derail your entire fitness journey.

So, how can you tell the difference between healthy workout soreness and potential injury pain? Well, here are some red flags to watch out for:

Sharp pain: This is a clear sign that something isn't right. Don't ignore it!

Pain that worsens with activity: If the pain gets worse during or after exercise, it's a sign you need to rest and potentially consult a healthcare professional.

Pain that lingers: Muscle soreness typically fades within a day or two. If the pain persists for several days, it could be an injury.

Swelling or bruising: These can be indicators of a more serious issue and require medical attention.

Remember, you are your own best advocate. Don't be afraid to modify exercises, adjust the intensity, or take a rest day when your body needs it. There's no shame in listening to your body's signals – it's the key to preventing injuries and ensuring your fitness journey is sustainable in the long run.

Here are some additional tips for making rest and recovery a priority:

Prioritise sleep: Aim for 7-8 hours of quality sleep each night. During sleep, your body repairs and rebuilds itself, making it crucial for recovery.

Active recovery: On rest days, engage in low-impact activities like walking, yoga, or light stretching. This helps keep your blood flowing and promotes

Active recovery (continued): promotes healing while preventing stiffness.

Foam rolling and self-massage: As I mentioned earlier, foam rolling can be a lifesaver for tight muscles and improved range of motion. Spend 10-15 minutes focusing on major muscle groups like your quads, hamstrings, glutes, and calves.

Listen to your mood: Sometimes, fatigue or low energy levels can be signs your body needs a break. Don't force yourself into a workout if you're feeling drained – listen to your mood and prioritise rest if needed.

Schedule rest days: Just like you schedule your workouts, schedule rest days into your routine. Treat them with the same importance as your workout sessions.

Cross-training: This involves incorporating different types of exercise into your routine. For example, if you typically do bodyweight workouts, consider adding a yoga or Pilates session to your week. This helps prevent overuse injuries and keeps things interesting.

By incorporating these strategies into your routine, you can make rest and recovery an essential part of your fitness journey. Remember, it's not just about the grind and the burn – it's about creating a sustainable, healthy relationship with exercise. Listen to your body, prioritise recovery, and watch your fitness journey flourish!

Now, let's talk about the mental aspect of listening to your body. This challenge has been a rollercoaster of emotions, just like any fitness journey.   There were days when I felt like a total rockstar, conquering those workouts with a smile

on my face.   But there were also days when the thought of another lunge made me groan internally. Those days, it wasn't just my muscles that needed a break – my mind did too.

That's when I discovered the importance of "mind-body connection". Taking the time to listen to how my body was feeling also meant acknowledging my mental state. If I was feeling stressed or overwhelmed, forcing myself into a gruelling workout wouldn't do any good. In those situations, I learned to prioritise activities that calmed my mind and reduced stress. Maybe it was a relaxing yoga session in the park, a long walk in nature, or simply some meditation before bed. Focusing on my mental well-being helped me return to my workouts feeling refreshed and motivated.

Remember, exercise is about more than just physical fitness – it's about overall well-being. So, listen to your body, not just physically, but mentally as well. Create a workout routine that complements your mental state and allows you to show up feeling your best, both physically and mentally.

Here's the thing: This journey isn't over. The beauty of bodyweight workouts is that they're versatile and adaptable. As I continue to progress, I can explore more advanced variations, increase the intensity, or add weight (think weighted vests or backpacks) to challenge myself further. But one thing remains constant: listening to my body. It's the compass that will guide me towards sustainable progress, prevent injuries, and ensure that this

A fitness journey is not just rewarding, but also enjoyable in the long run.

So, my fellow fitness enthusiasts, remember this: Your body is your temple. Treat it with respect, listen to its signals, and prioritise rest and recovery. Embrace the journey, celebrate the victories, and enjoy the process of becoming a stronger, healthier, and happier you! Now, get out there and move your body!

PART IV

Beyond Bodyweight Exercises

"Activities for a Well-Rounded Routine"

Conquered those push-ups and lunges? Feeling awesome (you should!), but craving a little more variety? That's where this chapter comes in! Think of bodyweight exercises as a fantastic foundation, but your fitness journey can be so much more! This chapter is your launchpad into a world of exciting activities that will keep your workouts fresh, challenge your body in new ways, and keep that fitness fire burning bright.

CHAPTER 17

Low-Impact Activities

"Walking, Swimming, Yoga for Older Adults"

Alright, champions! We've explored the wonders of bodyweight exercises, ventured beyond them with a variety of activities, and now it's time to delve into the world of low-impact exercises. Here's the thing – low-impact doesn't mean low-benefit! These activities are gentle on your joints but offer a powerful punch when it comes to boosting your fitness, improving your health, and keeping you feeling your best.

Whether you're a seasoned fitness enthusiast or just starting your journey, low-impact exercises are fantastic for everyone. They're perfect for older adults looking to maintain mobility and strength, individuals recovering from injuries, or anyone who wants to reap the benefits of exercise without the pounding impact of high-intensity workouts. So, grab your water bottle, strap on your comfy shoes, and let's explore some low-impact powerhouses!

Walking :

Let's start with a classic – walking! There's a reason it's called "man's (and woman's!) best exercise." Walking is accessible, requires minimal equipment (comfortable shoes are key!), and offers a plethora of benefits:

Improves cardiovascular health: A brisk walk gets your heart rate up, strengthens your heart muscle, and boosts overall cardiovascular health.

Maintains strength and mobility: Walking works various muscle groups, including your legs, core, and glutes. It also helps maintain joint mobility and flexibility.

 Get Fit and Feel Great

Weight management: Walking burns calories, which can aid in weight management or maintaining a healthy weight.

Stress reduction: A brisk walk in nature can be incredibly calming and stress-relieving. Fresh air and a change of scenery can do wonders for your mental well-being.

Start slow and gradually increase: If you're new to walking, begin with short distances and gradually increase the duration and intensity as your fitness improves.

Find a walking buddy: Having a friend or family member join you can make walking more enjoyable and motivating. You can chat, catch up, and support each other on your fitness journey.

Explore different terrains: Walking on different surfaces like trails, sidewalks, or even the beach can add a fun challenge and keep your walks interesting.

Set goals: Setting goals can help you stay motivated. Aim for a specific number of steps per day, a certain walking distance, or a specific time you want to spend walking.

Swimming:

Imagine feeling weightless, gliding through cool water, and getting a full-body workout – that's the magic of swimming! This low-impact activity is fantastic for people of all ages and fitness levels:

Full-body workout: Swimming engages all major muscle groups, promoting strength, endurance, and flexibility. It's a fantastic option for cross-training and giving your body a well-rounded workout.

Gentle on joints: The water's buoyancy takes the pressure off your joints, making it a perfect exercise for those with joint pain or injuries.

Improves cardiovascular health: Swimming gets your heart rate up and strengthens your cardiovascular system. It's a low-impact way to boost your cardio fitness.

Stress reduction: The rhythmic movements of swimming can be incredibly calming and stress-relieving.

Taking the Plunge:
Find a pool: This one's obvious, but joining a local pool or gym with a pool opens up a world of swimming possibilities.

Start with basic strokes: If you're new to swimming, focus on mastering basic strokes like the freestyle or breaststroke. You can always enrol in swimming lessons for proper technique.

Join a water aerobics class: These group classes offer a fun and dynamic way to exercise in the water. They incorporate various exercises, music, and social interaction to keep your workouts engaging.

Water walking: This is another fantastic low-impact option that's gentle on your joints but offers a great workout.

Yoga:
Yoga is more than just fancy poses on a mat. It's a holistic practice that combines physical postures (asanas), breathing exercises (pranayama), and meditation, offering a multitude of benefits:

Improves flexibility and mobility:* Yoga poses help lengthen and stretch your muscles, improving your overall flexibility and range of motion.

Builds strength and core stability:* Many yoga poses engage various muscle groups, promoting strength and core stability.

Reduces stress and anxiety: The focus on breath and mindful movements in yoga can be incredibly calming and help manage stress and anxiety.

Improves balance: Yoga poses challenges to your balance and coordination, which can improve stability and prevent falls, especially important for older adults.

Boosts mood and well-being: The combination of physical activity, mindfulness, and breathwork in

Yoga can leave you feeling energised, refreshed, and with a positive outlook.

Finding Your Yoga Flow:

Don't be intimidated: Yoga is for everyone, regardless of age or fitness level. Many yoga studios offer beginner classes specifically designed for those new to the practice.

Focus on proper form: Having a good foundation in yoga is crucial. Look for a certified yoga instructor who can guide you through poses with proper alignment to avoid injury.

Listen to your body: Yoga is not about pushing yourself to the limit. Modify poses as needed, and don't hesitate to take breaks when needed. Your comfort and safety are paramount.

Explore different styles: There are many different yoga styles, from the gentle and restorative to the more vigorous Vinyasa flow. Experiment with different styles to find what resonates most with you.

Low-impact exercises like walking, swimming, and yoga offer a multitude of benefits for people of all ages and fitness levels. Whether you're looking to maintain mobility, improve your cardiovascular health, reduce stress, or simply move your body in a gentle way, these activities are fantastic options.

CHAPTER 18

Staying Active Throughout the Day

"Incorporating Movement into Your Daily Life"

Alright, team! We've explored bodyweight workouts, ventured into different activities, and discovered the power of low-impact exercises. But what if your schedule feels like a never-ending to-do list, leaving little time for dedicated workouts? Fear not, fellow fitness warriors! This chapter is dedicated to showing you how to sneak movement into your daily life – little bursts of activity that add up throughout the day and keep you energised and active.

Let's face it, life can get hectic. Between work, family, errands, and the ever-present lure of the couch, carving out dedicated workout time can feel like a challenge. But the good news is, you don't need to spend hours at the gym to reap the benefits of exercise. Even small bursts of movement sprinkled throughout your day can make a significant difference. Here's how to become a master of the "movement-snack":

The Power of Micro-Workouts:
Think of micro-workouts as tiny bursts of activity – like bite-sized snacks for your body. They might not be a full-blown gym session, but these quick bursts of movement can get your blood pumping, improve your mood, and keep your body energised.

Here are some micro-workout ideas you can incorporate throughout your day:

Commercial Breaks: Don't waste those precious commercial breaks glued to the couch! Use them for some quick squats, lunges, jumping jacks, or push-ups. Even a few minutes of activity can make a difference.

Deskercise: Let's face it, sitting all day is the enemy of movement. Turn your desk into a mini-gym! Do some calf raises while checking emails, squeeze in some arm circles during a call, or perform some desk push-ups to strengthen your upper body.

The Parking Lot Shuffle: Instead of parking right next to the entrance, park farther away and walk those extra steps. It might seem insignificant, but those extra steps add up!

The Stairway Shuffle: Take the stairs whenever possible! Skip the elevator and climb those stairs – your legs and heart will thank you for it.

The Power of Cleaning: Turn your cleaning routine into a mini-workout. Crank up some music, move with intention as you clean, and turn mundane chores into a calorie-burning activity.

Making Movement a Habit:
The key to success with micro-workouts is consistency. Aim to incorporate these little bursts of movement throughout your day, making them a regular part of your routine. Here are some tips to help you make movement a habit:

Set reminders: Use your phone's alarm or a calendar notification to remind yourself to get up and move every hour.

Find a workout buddy: Enlist a friend, coworker, or family member to join you in your micro-workout adventures. Having someone to hold you accountable can be incredibly motivating.

Track your progress: Use a fitness tracker or a simple journal to track your daily movement. Seeing your progress can be a great motivator to keep going.

Make it fun! Put on some upbeat music, watch a funny video while doing jumping jacks, or find ways to make these micro-workouts enjoyable. The more fun you have, the more likely you are to stick with them.

Beyond Micro-Workouts:

Micro-workouts are fantastic, but incorporating movement into your daily life goes beyond quick bursts of activity. Here are some additional strategies to consider:

Active Errands: Can you walk or bike to your next errand instead of driving? How about scheduling a lunch break walk with a colleague? Find opportunities to be active even while completing your daily tasks.

Take the Active Commute: If your commute allows, walk, bike, or take public transportation (and walk those extra steps!). It's a great way to integrate movement into your daily routine.

Join a Sports League: Consider joining a recreational sports league (volleyball, soccer, badminton) – a fun and social way to get your body moving.

Active Family Time: Instead of a movie night, go for a family walk, play active games outdoors, or take a dance class together. Make active entertainment a part of your family time.

A dedicated workout routine is fantastic, but don't underestimate the power of incorporating movement throughout your day. These "sneaky" bursts of activity can play a significant role in boosting your energy levels, improving your mood, and keeping you fit and healthy. So, get creative, find ways to move your body throughout the day, and remember – every step counts!

CHAPTER 19

Finding a Fitness Buddy or Joining a Group Exercise Class

Remember Week Six of the bodyweight challenge? The one with those brutal burpees? Let's just say, staring at my living room wall while doing burpees wasn't exactly motivating. My form was suffering, my enthusiasm was dwindling, and I seriously considered calling it quits. Then, inspiration struck – a gym membership offer landed in my mailbox. Now, I'm not one for crowded gyms, but one phrase in the ad caught my eye – "Free Intro Week to Group Fitness Classes." Boom! That was the sign I needed.

The next week, I found myself stepping into a Zumba class, feeling a mix of nervousness and excitement. And guess what? It was exhilarating! The energy in the room was contagious, the instructor was fantastic, and suddenly, those burpees (incorporated into the Zumba routine, might I add!) felt more like a playful challenge than a dreaded exercise. That was the day I discovered the magic of group fitness classes.

The Buddy System:
Accountability: A workout buddy holds you accountable. Knowing someone is waiting for you at the gym or park can be a powerful motivator to show up and get moving.

Motivation and Support: A good buddy can be your biggest cheerleader! They'll motivate you to push your limits, celebrate your victories, and offer a shoulder to lean on during tough workouts.

Double the Fun: Working out with a friend can be a lot more fun than going solo. You can chat, laugh, and support each other throughout your workout.

Finding Your Perfect Match:

Reach out to your friends/family: Do you have a friend or family member who shares your fitness goals? Reach out and see if they'd be interested in joining you for workouts.

Social media groups: Join online fitness groups in your area. You might just find a like-minded individual looking for a workout buddy!

Gym or fitness centre: Many gyms offer buddy programs or boards where you can connect with other fitness enthusiasts.

The Wonderful World of Group Fitness Classes:

Now, let's talk about group fitness classes! Here's how they can benefit you:

Variety is the spice of life: With so many group fitness class options available (Zumba, yoga, HIIT, spinning, and more!), you'll never get bored. There's something for everyone!

Expert guidance: Group classes are led by certified instructors who can guide you through proper form and offer modifications if needed.

Motivation and Community: The energy in a group fitness class is infectious! You'll be surrounded by positive vibes and people working towards similar goals.

Finding Your Perfect Class:

With so many options, finding the right group fitness class might feel overwhelming. Here's how to navigate the choices:

Consider your interests: Do you enjoy upbeat music and dancing? Try Zumba or HIIT. Are you looking for something more calming? Yoga or Pilates might be a good fit.

Check out free intro classes: Many gyms offer free intro classes to different fitness classes. This is a fantastic way to try different options before committing to a specific class.

Don't be afraid to ask: Instructors and gym staff are there to help! Ask them for recommendations based on your fitness level and goals.

After that initial Zumba class, I was hooked! I started exploring different classes, discovering a newfound love for yoga and the challenge of HIIT workouts. The friends I made in those classes were an unexpected bonus. We became a little fitness support group, motivating each other, sharing healthy recipes, and even planning fun group activities outside the gym. There was a sense of community and camaraderie that I didn't expect, and it made the whole fitness journey even more enjoyable.

Whether you choose to find a workout buddy or join a group fitness class, surrounding yourself with others on your fitness journey can be incredibly beneficial. The accountability, motivation, and sense of community can make working out more enjoyable, help you stay on track, and even push you to achieve new levels of fitness. So, step outside your comfort zone, give it a try, and discover the power of working out with others!

PART VII

Resources and Tools for Your Bodyweight Exercise Journey

Imagine having access to free resources, handy apps, and inspiring workout routines – all designed to supercharge your bodyweight workouts. That's exactly what awaits you here. Get ready to unlock a treasure trove of tools that will keep you motivated, informed, and progressing on your path to fitness glory! Buckle up, because with the right resources at your fingertips, your bodyweight workouts are about to reach a whole new level! Let's unleash your inner fitness rockstar!

CHAPTER 20

Additional Resources

"Online Resources, Fitness Apps, and Support Groups"

WEBSITES: The internet is brimming with fantastic websites dedicated to bodyweight exercises. These sites offer exercise tutorials, workout routines, progressions for different fitness levels, and valuable information on proper form and technique. Here are a few to get you started:

- ACE Library of Exercises: URL ace library of exercises ON ACE Fitness acefitness.org
- The National Strength and Conditioning Association (NSCA): URL strength and

 Get Fit and Feel Great

conditioning ON National Strength and Conditioning Association nsca.com
- Darebee: URL darebee com
- YouTube Channels: YouTube is a haven for fitness enthusiasts! Numerous channels offer free bodyweight workout videos led by certified trainers. You'll find high-quality tutorials, follow-along workouts for all fitness levels, and energising routines to keep your workouts exciting. Here are a few popular channels:
- Fitness Blender
- Chloe Ting
- MadFit

FITNESS APPS:

Fitness apps can be fantastic companions on your bodyweight journey. They offer a variety of features to keep you on track, including:

Workout routines: Many apps provide pre-designed bodyweight workout routines that cater to different fitness levels and goals.

Exercise tutorials: Get clear video demonstrations and instructions for proper form and technique.

Progression tracking: Track your progress over time and see how you're improving with each workout.

Community features: Some apps offer social features that allow you to connect with other fitness enthusiasts, share your experiences, and stay motivated.

Here are a few popular fitness apps to consider:
- Nike Training Club
- Sworkit
- FitOn
- JEFIT

SUPPORT GROUPS:

Feeling the need for some extra encouragement and a sense of community? Look no further than online support groups! These groups can be a fantastic source of motivation, information, and camaraderie. Here are a few ways to find supportive communities:

Facebook Groups: Search for groups dedicated to bodyweight exercises, fitness motivation, or your specific fitness goals.

Online Forums: Many fitness websites have forums where you can connect with other exercisers, ask questions, and share your experiences.

Local Meetups: Look for bodyweight exercise groups or fitness clubs in your area. Working out with others can add a fun social element and keep you accountable.

APPENDIX A

Sample Bodyweight Exercise Routines for Different Fitness Levels

These are just samples. Feel free to adjust the exercises, sets, reps, and rest periods based on your own fitness level and goals. It's crucial to listen to your body, take rest days when needed, and gradually increase intensity as you get stronger.

Warm-Up is Key!
Before diving into any workout, a proper warm-up is crucial. Aim for 5-10 minutes of light cardio like jumping jacks, jogging on the spot, or arm circles to get your blood flowing and muscles warmed up.

Don't skip this step – it helps prevent injuries and prepares your body for the workout ahead.

Cool Down and Stretch Don't Forget!

After your workout, don't just collapse on the couch! Dedicate 5-10 minutes to cooling down with some light cardio and static stretches. This helps your body recover properly and prevents muscle soreness.

Ready, Set, Bodyweight Blast Off!

Here are your sample bodyweight exercise routines:

Beginner Routine (Focus on Form and Technique): This routine focuses on mastering basic bodyweight exercises with proper form. Aim for 2-3 sets of 10-15 repetitions for each exercise, with 30 seconds rest between sets.

Squats: This classic exercise works your legs and core. Stand with your feet shoulder-width apart, toes slightly outward. Lower your body as if sinking into a chair, keeping your back straight and core engaged. Push through your heels to stand back up.

Push-ups (Modified): If regular push-ups are challenging, start with modified push-ups. Perform them on your knees, keeping your back straight and core engaged. Lower your chest towards the ground and press back up.

Lunges: This exercise works your legs and glutes. Step forward with one leg, lowering your body down until both knees are bent at 90-degree angles. Push through your front heel to return to standing. Repeat with the other leg.

Plank: This exercise strengthens your core and back. Lie on your stomach with your forearms on the ground, elbows shoulder-width apart. Keep your body in a straight line from head to heels, engaging your core muscles. Hold for 30 seconds.

Rest: Take 30 seconds of rest before repeating the circuit.

Intermediate Routine (Challenge Yourself!):
This routine builds upon the basic exercises, increasing difficulty and intensity. Aim for 3 sets of 12-15 repetitions for each exercise, with 30 seconds rest between sets.

Squats with Jump: Perform a regular squat, and as you stand up, jump explosively. Land softly and immediately go into the next squat.

Push-ups: If modified push-ups were a breeze, try regular push-ups! Keep your form strict – back straight, core engaged, and lower your chest towards the ground.

Walking Lunges: Take a lunge with one leg, walk forward with that same leg, and then lunge with the other leg. This keeps your heart rate elevated and adds an extra challenge.

Side Plank: Similar to a plank, but on one side. Prop yourself up on one forearm, with your body in a straight line from head to heels. Engage your core and hold for 30 seconds per side.

Rest: Take 30 seconds of rest before repeating the circuit.

Advanced Routine (Push Your Limits!):
This routine is designed for those who are already comfortable with bodyweight exercises and are looking for a serious challenge. Aim for 3 sets of

8-10 repetitions for each exercise, with 45 seconds rest between sets.

Pistol Squats: This single-leg squat variation requires balance and strength. Stand on one leg and lower your body down until your other leg nearly touches the ground. Push through your heel to stand back up. Repeat with the other leg.

Diamond Push-ups: These push-ups require closer hand placement, targeting your triceps. Place your hands close together, forming a diamond shape with your thumbs and index fingers. Lower your chest towards the ground and press back up.

Bulgarian Split Squats: Similar to lunges, but performed with your back foot elevated on a bench or chair. This adds extra difficulty for your quads and glutes.

Mountain Climbers: This exercise gets your heart rate up and works your core and legs. Start in a high plank position, then alternate bringing your knees towards your chest in a running motion.

Rest: Take 45 seconds of rest before repeating the circuit.

With dedication, consistency, and the right tools, you can achieve amazing results with bodyweight exercises. So, lace up your sneakers, grab your water bottle, and get ready to conquer your fitness goals!

APPENDIX B

Glossary of Exercise Terms

Aerobic Exercise:

Exercises that get your heart rate up and keep it elevated for a sustained period, promoting efficient oxygen use. Examples include brisk walking, swimming, and cycling. (Introduced in Chapter 1)

Bodyweight Exercise:

Exercises that use your own body weight as resistance. Examples include squats, push-ups, lunges, and planks. (Introduced in Chapter 1)

Calorie:

A unit of energy used to measure the energy burned during exercise and the energy provided by food. (Introduced in Chapter 2)

Core:

The group of muscles that support your spine and pelvis, including your abs, obliques, and lower back. (Introduced in Chapter 2)

Form:

The proper technique for performing an exercise. Maintaining good form is crucial to prevent injury and maximise effectiveness.

High-intensity Interval Training (Hiit):

Short bursts of intense exercise followed by periods of rest or low-intensity activity. (Introduced in Chapter 4)

Isometric Exercise:

Exercises that involve contracting a muscle without moving a joint. Examples include planks and wall sits. (Introduced in Chapter 5)

Modification:

Adapting an exercise to make it easier or more challenging, depending on your fitness level or limitations. (Introduced in Appendix B)

Muscle Group

A group of muscles that work together to perform a specific movement. Examples include quadriceps (thighs), hamstrings (back of thighs), and biceps (upper arms). (Introduced in Chapter 2)

Repetition (Rep):

One complete performance of an exercise. (Introduced in Chapter 2)

Rest Period:

The time you take between sets of exercises to allow your body to recover. (Introduced in Chapter 2)

Set:

A group of repetitions performed consecutively. (Introduced in Chapter 2)

Strength Training:

Exercises that aim to build muscle strength and endurance. Bodyweight exercises like squats, lunges, and push-ups are all forms of strength training. (Introduced in Chapter 1)

Warm-up:

Light cardio and dynamic stretches performed before a workout to prepare your body for exercise and prevent injury. (Introduced in Appendix A)

Cool-down:

Light cardio and static stretches performed after a workout to help your body recover and prevent muscle soreness. (Introduced in Appendix A)

CONCLUSION

Congratulations! You've reached the culmination of this guide, and by doing so, you've taken a significant step towards a healthier and more fulfilling future. The knowledge and tools you've acquired here serve as the foundation for a sustainable lifestyle that prioritises your well-being. Celebrate each milestone, big or small, and never lose sight of the incredible strength and resilience you possess.

Remember, this journey is not about achieving an unattainable ideal; it's about steady and meaningful progress. There may be days when motivation wanes, but that's simply a natural part of the process. During those times, draw upon the knowledge and strategies outlined within these pages, and know that there's a supportive community (myself included!) rooting for your success.

Most importantly, find joy in the process. Embrace the invigorating power of movement, rediscover the remarkable capabilities of your body, and live your life to the fullest. Remember, you, remarkable woman, deserve to feel your absolute best. Now, go forth and conquer your goals with confidence and a renewed sense of vitality!